Nursing Careers

Easily Choose What Nursing Career Will Make Your 12 Hour Shift a Blast!

Chase Hassen
Nurse Superhero
© 2016

Disclaimer:

Although the author and publisher have made every effort to ensure that the information in this book was correct at press time, the author and publisher do not assume and hereby disclaim any liability to any party for any loss, damage, or disruption caused by errors or omissions, whether such errors or omissions result from negligence, accident, or any other cause.

This book is not intended as a substitute for the medical advice of physicians. The reader should regularly consult a physician in matters relating to his/her health and particularly with respect to any symptoms that may require diagnosis or medical attention.

All rights reserved. No part of this publication may be reproduced, distributed, or transmitted in any form or by any means, including photocopying, recording, or other electronic or mechanical methods, without the prior written permission of the publisher, except in the case of brief quotations embodied in critical reviews and certain other noncommercial uses permitted by copyright law.

NCLEX®, NCLEX®-RN, and NCLEX®-PN are registered trademarks of the National Council of State Boards of Nursing, Inc. They hold no affiliation with this product.

First, I want to give you this FREE gift...

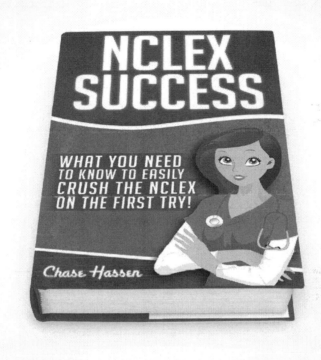

For a limited time, you can download this book for FREE.

Visit this website below:

bit.ly/NclexSuccessDownloadNow

Table of Contents

Chapter 1:

Introduction to an RN Career

Nursing is an area of medicine in which there is the great potential for job growth. Registered nurses must complete a four year post-high school education and pass an exam that leads to a registered nursing degree. From there, you can work as a registered nurse or continue on to post-graduate nursing fields such as nurse midwifery, Master's degree in nursing, nurse anaesthetist, clinical nurse specialist, or nurse practitioner.

As a registered nurse, you can work in clinical medicine in a hospital or clinic, as a flight nurse, a school nurse, home health nurse or a cruise ship nurse, among others. You can also work in non-clinical settings, such as in nursing education, community nursing educator, nursing education and clinical research. In short, there are many pathways that lead from the four year program to a wide range of nursing jobs.

Nurses are a respected member of the healthcare team and have a great deal of responsibility when it comes to taking care of, following the progress of, and educating patients and their families in a variety of healthcare situations. As a registered nurse, you can work relatively independently or work as part of a healthcare team that cares for and educates patients.

There are numerous specialty options when it comes to using your degree. For example, as a hospital nurse, you can subspecialize in some of the following areas:

Emergency medicine

Critical care

Hospice care

Labor and delivery

Neonatal care

Oncology

OR nursing

Dialysis care

Staff nursing

You can also work as an outpatient nurse in school systems, as a home health nurse, as a flight nurse, a clinic nurse, a nursing home nurse or even as a cruise ship nurse. As you can see, being a registered nurse is different for everyone and there are many areas you can work in. Registered nurses make on average approximately $65,000 per year with compensation depending on your level of education, geographic location, the type of facility you work in, and your experience level. If you have an advanced degree along with your education as a registered nurse, you can easily make in excess of $80,000 per year.

You will go through less unnecessary education if you make a decision as to the area of nursing you want to go into before you complete your degree. That way, you can focus on those areas most applicable to getting the kind of education you need before graduating. The purpose of this book is to help you decide what kind of nursing most appeals to you as a registered nurse. As you read this book, try to decide which areas you would most like to work in and direct your education accordingly.

Chapter 2:

Hospital Nursing

RNs make up the bulk of nurses working in hospital settings. In smaller hospitals, you may find yourself taking care of a wide variety of patients, from general ward patients, to post-operative patients, to labor and delivery patients. In larger hospitals, many nurses work in specialized areas as noted in chapter 1. There are a variety of subspecialties you might find yourself drawn to as a hospital nurse. Let's look at some of these subspecialties:

Emergency medicine. You work in an emergency department, seeing patients who have a wide variety of problems that bring them to the hospital. An emergency room nurse needs to know about many different areas of medicine and must understand the rules of triaging patients. In triage, you take care of the more critical patients before caring for those who have minor injuries. The patients you see come off the streets of their own accord or by ambulance and it is a challenge to identify what's wrong with the patient and direct their care to the community, the hospital, or to a clinic for follow up. You must work with emergency medicine doctors who are trained similarly to the way you were trained—to deal with whatever comes in the door.

Critical care. In critical care nursing, you work in the Intensive Care Unit with patients who are the sickest patients in the hospital. In large facilities, you will work with a hospitalist, who specializes in caring for hospitalized patients. You will need to understand complex aspects of ventilator care, the care of the cardiac patient, and the care of sick patients who have recently had surgery. Often, you will care for only one or two patients at a time that need round the clock intensive care.

Hospice care. This involves caring for patients who are in the active process of dying and who are expected to live no longer than six months. This can involve caring for these patients in a hospital setting or in a home setting, where the goal of care is palliative rather than curative. In hospice care, you will care for a variety of patients, including patients with cancer and other terminal illnesses. In hospice care, the focus is on keeping the patient as comfortable as possible while they are in the dying process.

Labor and delivery. In this part of the hospital, you will care for laboring mothers who are trying to have their baby vaginally and will assist the doctor in managing the labor and delivery. You may also take part in Cesarean sections as a scrub nurse or as the nurse caring for the infant once it is born. Regardless of the method of delivery, you will care for the postpartum patient and help her care for her infant. You will educate the mother and family on infant care and on postpartum care of the mother. Mothers do not stay in the hospital as long as they used to, so you must pack a lot of education into a short period of time.

Neonatal care. If an infant is born prematurely or is born with some kind of anomaly or illness, they are taken care of in a special part of the hospital called the neonatal intensive care unit. This is a challenging area of pediatric medicine in which you need to know a great deal about the medications and specialty care given to very tiny patients and their families. In the case of premature infants and very sick infants, you may have the same patient for many weeks as they grow and get better from whatever is ailing them. This involves a lot of parental education as well as very particular cares given to very fragile patients.

Oncology. As an oncology nurse, you deal exclusively with cancer patients. Many of these patients are in the hospital receiving chemotherapy. Above all nurses, you understand the intricacies of chemotherapy and other medical/surgical modalities for cancer care. Patients with cancer are often in and out of the hospital, depending on their response to their treatment and you may deal with them as an outpatient as well. Oncology nurses often work closely with hospice staff as not every patient with cancer will recover and some will require transfer to a hospice setting.

OR nursing. Operating room nurses work with the patient before, during and/or after surgery. As an operating room nurse, you understand the intricacies of working in a sterile setting, assisting surgeons in a variety of settings and working with the anesthetist or anesthesiologist in the care of the patient undergoing surgery. These patients need an extensive workup prior to having surgery and nurses do a lot of this type of work to make sure the patient is ready for surgery. Other RNs can work with patients in recovery, who are awakening from anesthesia and need special attention as well as instructions for going home or to another part of the hospital for care.

Dialysis care. This can be done in a hospital setting or at a specialized dialysis center where patients with chronic kidney failure receive dialysis on a regular basis. This requires an extensive knowledge of nephrology and of the various diseases a patient can get that results in the need for dialysis. Dialysis is a specialty procedure requiring skilled knowledge and nursing skills.

Staff nursing. As a staff nurse, you work with patients who have a variety of illnesses but are not sick enough to require specialty care. The general ward usually treats adults although you can specialize in treating children on a special pediatric wing of the hospital. You help care for the patients daily needs, give medications, and help them transition from the hospital to a nursing facility or to home care.

Working in a hospital generally means you spend 8-12 hours working at any given shift. You may work primarily during the days, in the evenings or during the night shift. Many nurses pick a certain shift and stick with it, while others take day and/or night shifts as they come up.

Chapter 3:

Outpatient Clinic Careers

As a nurse in an outpatient clinic, you have a variety of jobs to do. In some cases, you are the liaison between the patient calling with questions and the doctor who doesn't have the time to answer every phone call that comes into the clinic. You are responsible for medical records and helping the doctor manage patients who call into the clinic. This can involve dealing with pharmacy requests by phone or fax as well.

As a clinic nurse, you may be supervising medical assistants or you may take patients to their outpatient clinic room yourself. You are responsible for keeping the patients' medication and allergy lists up to date and you help manage the medical records. As an RN, you may assist on outpatient procedures such as suturing, specialty examinations, and treatments.

You may practice at a family practice, internal medicine, pediatric, or specialty clinic in which your jobs may vary widely. Every doctor has a different sort of practice, depending on their specialty so you may need to be trained regarding the different procedures the doctors you work for specialize in. For example, if you work in a urology clinic, you may assist the doctor in the performance of cystoscopy examinations as well as other clinic duties. If you work in a colorectal surgeon's clinic, you may assist him or her in doing outpatient colonoscopies or proctoscopies. This can involve giving sedating medications and following patient vital signs during the various procedures.

You can work at an outpatient surgical center. In this case, many different minor surgeries are done in a freestanding clinic. Because it is a surgical center, your job description may match the job description of a hospital OR nurse, with the exception that the patients usually go home following their surgery. Even so, they need preoperative evaluation, operating room care, and postoperative monitoring, along with postoperative instructions and follow up care. The difference between you and a hospital OR nurse is that the procedures you help the doctor with tend to be more minor with the expectation that the patient will awaken from surgery and will be able to go home with education from you and the doctor as to postoperative care and follow up. You generally work days, although the day may start very early in the morning and go throughout the afternoon.

If you work in a pediatric clinic, you help check in child patients and get ready to see the doctor. You are trained in the medications, illnesses and vital signs of sick and healthy children and you are trained in giving vaccinations. You work with the doctor on procedures done as an outpatient and you educate parents when it comes to caring for their children.

Caring for patients in an outpatient setting usually means you work an 8 am to 5 pm job, Mondays through Fridays, with the possibility of some Saturday work. If you work in an urgent care clinic, the hours may be extended, involving the care of patients in the early to late evening hours, including weekends. Urgent care clinics are outpatient clinics that handle a variety of patients with minor problems not severe enough to require a visit to the emergency department. There are some urgent care clinics operating within hospitals or as free-standing clinics. It is a little bit like working in an emergency department in that you don't have the same patients coming back over and over again and you likely won't do as much telephone consultation work as you would if you worked in a regular outpatient clinic. You may also be assisting in minor procedures such as suturing of minor wounds or helping with splints and crutches.

Chapter 4:

Flight Nursing

With a little extra training and a certification, you can find yourself in the exciting world of flight nursing. Flight nurses have special training in giving medical care during the transportation of a patient by air—either through a helicopter flight or through flight with a fixed-wing airplane. Many of these flights carry extremely ill patients requiring emergency transport following a severe automobile accident or following basic medical care at a small rural hospital that doesn't have the capabilities of caring for anyone who is as ill as the patient is. Besides skills in emergency nursing, flight nurses need to develop skills in flight and navigation.

Flight nurses can work in the military or as a civilian. Civilian flight nurses have a greater ability to choose where it is they would like to work but military flight nurses generally make a far greater salary. The disadvantages of working in the military sector is that you generally have to work overseas in a war torn area, extracting seriously ill and wounded patients from dangerous areas.

Fight nurses may actually take part in some of the flight responsibilities if patient responsibilities are not necessary. This can include taking part in navigation and radio communication. Generally they begin by following the instructions of the sending physician, if there is one, or by following generally accepted emergency medicine procedures if the patient is being transferred from an accident scene. Contact is generally made with an emergency medical physician at the destination site, who will give orders based on your assessment of the patient. There will often be paperwork that needs to be carefully kept on board the aircraft. This paperwork is the responsibility of the flight nurse as well as the paramedics or physicians on board until you reach your destination facility.

When patients are transferred from an accident or other trauma, basic trauma life support techniques are used by the transport team, including the flight nurse. Patients need to be secured to a gurney inside the helicopter or fixed-wing aircraft because the flight can involve turbulence or jostling around of the patient.

The various activities done on the flight can include resuscitation measures, based on advanced trauma life support protocols, the starting of IVs if necessary and the use of other advanced life support procedures. If there is contact with a destination emergency physician, you will follow the doctor's orders after giving them continual update as to the condition of the patient. This is generally a very frightening time for the patient, so he or she will need constant reassurance that they are being taken care of.
Flight nurses, along with paramedics, are responsible for transferring the critically ill patient from the helicopter or fixed wing aircraft to the destination hospital. It can mean

landing on the roof of the hospital or a nearby helipad or airport with transfer to the hospital via an additional ambulance transfer. Paperwork is filled out and transferred along with the patient, which updates the receiving facility as to the various things that happened at the sending facility and enroute to the receiving hospital.

Flight nurses do most of their work thousands of feet in the air in a cramped helicopter or in a small, fixed wing airplane. If you work as a civilian flight nurse, you are usually employed by a trauma center or large hospital that has helicopters that fly to other hospitals or to accident scenes, depending on need. You can also work for an independent medical evacuation corporation, a search and rescue organization, or a fire department.

As a military flight nurse, you usually belong to a branch of the US military, including reserve military units. Most commonly, you will work overseas where the US has a military base that has a military hospital set up and in which there is war going on.

In order to become a flight nurse, you need to earn your four year nursing degree and pass the NCLEX-RN examination (the National Council Licensure Examination for Registered Nurses Examination). You then pursue training as an emergency nurse or as an intensive care nurse. After gaining experience on the ground, you can study and take the Certified Flight Registered Nurses Examination, which is a test offered to you by the Board of Certification for Emergency Nursing. After that you can work in the civilian sector as a flight nurse. You can also be trained by the military and gain experience in the field as a military flight nurse.

Chapter 5:

Cruise Ship Nursing

Every large cruise ship has a medical department for the treatment of passengers and crew who become ill or injured while the cruise ship is at sea. This is an exciting job in which you can travel to all parts of the world, depending on what cruise liner you work for. You will work with a physician or physicians, other nurses and possibly a nurse practitioner or paramedic. The size of the medical department depends on the size of the cruise ship and on the number of crew-members and passengers aboard the ship. Because you may take care of anything from minor to severe illnesses and injuries, you may need to be ATLS or ACLS certified so you can deal with advanced trauma or cardiovascular emergencies.

Because you will be gone for long periods of time, you may have nice accommodations including accommodations for your spouse or family, depending on the cruise line you work for. The ship, for all intents and purposes, is your home for as long as you have the job of working on the cruise ship.

If you have an advanced degree as a nurse practitioner, you work relatively independently as a nurse practitioner, seeing patients and performing administrative work in the cruise ship's medical clinic. Nurse practitioners can do many of the same things as doctors and work under the supervision of the lead physician on the cruise ship.

If you are working in the capacity as a ship nurse, you report to the head nurse or to the physicians at the ship's medical clinic. You need the following to be able to work effectively as a cruise ship nurse:

> You need to have a diploma from nursing school and be certified as a registered nurse.

> Ideally, you should have at least two to three years of clinical experience as an outpatient nurse or as an emergency room nurse.

> You should be certified in Basic Life Support and Advanced Cardiac Life Support (ACLS). Some cruise lines request Advanced Trauma Life Support (ATLS) certification as well.

> You may need to have experience in dealing with laboratory procedures and basic x-ray procedures as there is not likely to be a lab tech or x-ray tech on duty.

> You should have a background in general medicine and/or emergency medicine.

You should have past experience caring for patients in a trauma, cardiac care, emergency care, or internal medicine practice.

Because cruise liners travel to often to foreign lands and have people of all different cultures on board, you may need to have knowledge of other languages besides English.

As a cruise ship nurse, you work under the direction of the head nurse and physicians also working with you on the cruise ship caring for the day to day injuries and illnesses that come up as part of the care of patients, who may be staff members of the cruise ship or passengers.

You may be the initial contact the patient has, even before seeing the physician and you are responsible for gaining medical information, including medications, vital signs, and allergies the patient has. You may have to provide first aid to the patient until other staff members arrive on the scene of an illness or injury. You work much like an urgent care clinic, caring for patients with a variety of ailments, including things like sunburn, food poisoning, colds and flu, and minor illnesses. Some patients travel with serious underlying conditions that may have to be managed at sea.

The starting salary of a cruise ship nurse is about $4200-$4900 USD per month, with or without free accommodations and board. Your salary will be higher if you take on the lead or head nurse position.

Chapter 6:

Home Health Nursing

Home health nurse require a four year RN degree and the passage of the NCLEX-RN examination. You don't need to have any extra training—just the desire to work independently out of people's homes.

As a home health nurse, you manage the care of a patient who can't get out to seek medical care very often and who need services of a home healthcare team, usually led by the home health nurse. The home health nurse acts as a liaison between the patient and the doctor's clinic and is usually able to do things like urinalysis and blood draws on patients needing in-home evaluation. You can also be responsible for ordering home health aide services, physical therapy, and occupational therapy for the patient and may make referrals to services like meals-on-wheels for people with nutritional deficiencies and who can't cook meals for themselves.

You may work for a small or large home health agency with a salary of between $39,000 and $50,000 and you may be reimbursed for the gas you use while travelling from home to home.

Many of the people you work with are elderly who have limited mobility. You may also work for young children who have mobility or developmental issues. People who have recently had surgery or are discharged from the hospital may require a few weeks of home health services from an RN in order to follow their care at home before the patient can be independent.

The RN is usually responsible for managing the patient's medications, particularly if they have a lot of medication to take. Some people go home on oxygen or with post-operative drains that need the ongoing attention of an RN. You can specialize as an ostomy nurse, who handles people who have had an ileostomy or a colostomy and are just figuring out how to manage them. Wound infection devices and IV therapy can even be managed at home with the right home health nurse managing the care.

The RN who does home care often works with people on a long term basis; he or she is responsible for the home care plan that the patient and other members of the staff will follow. The goal of home health nursing is to try and get the patient to become as independent as possible; however, this might not ever happen, especially with the elderly and those with developmental disabilities.

As a home health nurse, your job will be multi-faceted and you will dabble in many different areas of medicine, including some hospice care, general medicine and nursing home care. Patients need a variety of things that can be done or ordered by the home health care nurse.

This is a job for a nurse who wants some independence and variety in his or her day. It is an important and necessary part of caring for patients from the time they are sick in the hospital until they become independent or die from their illness. While you are employed by a home health agency, many of the orders come directly from the patient's doctor. You will be working with many different doctors on a variety of patients who have different needs all the time.

This job is partly clinical and partly directed toward coordination of care. As a home health nurse, you will take vital signs, evaluate surgical wounds, change catheters, draw blood, or obtain urine samples, keeping track of the home-bound patient's healthcare as though you were part of the patient's clinic. With the advent of newer technologies, you may Instagram message a patient's wound or lesion directly to the doctor so as to keep the patient home as much as possible without having to see the doctor on an every day or every other day basis.

Chapter 7:

School Nursing

Nearly every school system has a school nursing program, which in many cases is just one RN who helps teachers and students manage health issues for the school system. Sometimes there is an RN for every school, while in smaller school systems, there is one or two nurses to cover for all students in the school district from elementary school through high school.

The school nurse works relatively independently in a small office that has an area for sick students to lie down on, a filing cabinet and nurse's desk. You will have the medical records and possibly the immunization records of all students and will care students that become ill at school while contacting the child's parents and/or doctor.

Emergencies can happen at school and the nurse often acts as first responder to these types of emergencies, such as falls in the playground, fights with injuries, and other injuries at school. Some of these injuries can be taken care of at school with the parents notified and the patient remaining at school, while at other times, you may care for the child until the parent(s) come to pick the child up. You may have to work with local paramedics if the situation warrants an ambulance transfer to the hospital.

The school nurse is also involved in health education of individual students with questions and on school-wide or district-wide health issues. You can work with parents and children on preventing community-transferred communicable diseases such as pediculosis (head lice), flu, and colds. There may be smoking and alcohol education issues in middle school and high school as well as issues regarding sexual intercourse and pregnancy prevention in high school students.

The school nurse must be sure that letters are sent out whenever there are communicable diseases such as pediculosis to parents of contacts with the index patient and may partake in screenings for pediculosis.

The school nurse has a wide variety of jobs to do that can range from mundane to life-threatening, depending on the day and the circumstances. As the school nurse, you are the go-to person for all health questions and issues raised in the course of a school day. You must be able to work relatively independently and with authority. There will be doctors to answer to in some cases, while in the vast majority of cases, you will work only with the parents, teachers and students on various health issues.

Chapter 8:

Locum Tenens Nursing

A locum tenens nurse is one who works for a locum tenens or "temp" agency directly working for the healthcare sector. As a locum tenens nurse, you get to choose where and when you get to work, and you can work in a wide variety of medical situations, based on your interest, education and background.

Locum tenens nurses are sort of like what "substitute teachers" are to" teachers". You work in situations where a hospital, clinic or nursing facility needs the temporary services of a registered nurse or are looking to try out a temporary nurse before hiring her full time. You are paid by the organization who you work for or from the temporary agency itself.

Because there is a big demand for locum tenens health professionals, you tend to make more money doing this than you would if you worked a regular RN position; however, your hours are not guaranteed and you might work a lot during any given week or month and not at all in the weeks or months to follow. There are usually no benefit packages such as health insurance or retirement funds so you are basically working for money for yourself and your family without any perks.

Locum tenens positions have a lot of advantages. You can set your own hours and can work in a variety of positions. It is a good job for starting nurses who don't yet know what kind of work they want to do and want to try different locations and job duties before selecting one that fits best for them. You can choose what kinds of areas of nursing you want to work as a locum tenens nurse in and can accept or turn down job offers as you wish. You are essentially your own employer and are free to do as you wish in order to earn an income.

Some of the downsides of working as a locum tenens position is that you don't have a steady income to count on, the drive times to work can be extensive, and you don't generally have any perks such as retirement and healthcare coverage. You don't work with the same people every time so the camaraderie among nurses is lacking in your workplace. You will be relatively unfamiliar with the standard practices of every place you work at so you may have to rely on the regular staff there when it comes to what the various protocols are. Nothing is consistent and things can quickly become quite difficult if you are in a situation where you need information you haven't been there long enough to have.

You can work as a locum tenens nurse while you are looking for a permanent position. It allows you to have an income while you are trying to find a permanent position. In some cases, the places you work for are using a locum tenens service because they can't find a full time staff person to work the position you are working in. In such cases, you are essentially "trying out" a job that you later can accept on a full time basis.

Chapter 9:

Advanced Nursing Degrees

Once you have your RN degree and pass the NCLEX-RN examination, you have the opportunity to further your education in several areas of advanced medicine. Most are essentially the equivalent of getting your Master's degree in a specialty area of your choosing. This chapter covers some of the areas you might select when furthering your nursing education.

Nurse Anesthetist

When you further your education to become a CRNA or Certified Nurse Anesthetist, you are choosing to become a specialized nurse who helps patients during anesthesia while they are having surgery. Certified nurse anesthetists practice throughout the US and administer anesthetics to patients about 35 million times per year.

In order to become a CRNA, you attend an accredited nurse anesthesia school receiving education that allows you to pass a national certification examination to become a CRNA. This involves both classroom and clinical education lasting an additional year or two beyond your four year college degree. You will learn many areas of medicine and biology, including coursework in chemistry, physics, pathophysiology, anatomy, physiology, pharmacology and anesthesia. You will learn the various clinical practices and procedures necessary to become capable of handling patients who are undergoing anesthesia during surgery or during obstetrical procedures.

The degree you get is the equivalent of a Master's degree, which can be in an allied health area, biological sciences, nursing and/or clinical sciences. In order to go for the program, you must have a Bachelor of Science degree in nursing or a related clinical program. You must carry an RN license by virtue of having passed the NCLEX-RN examination. Almost all programs require that you have at least one year of experience in acute care nursing. Financial aid is available for those who qualify as well as student loans in most cases.

As a CRNA, you will manage the care of the anesthesia before, during and after a patient has had surgery or during the delivery of a baby. You will perform physical assessments, teach the patient about anesthesia, prepare the patient for anesthesia, administer medications to keep the patient free of pain, keep the anesthesia going in the operating room, oversee the recovery of the patient from anesthesia and follow the patient's care until discharge from the surgery area. As a CRNA, you will work with doctors, surgeons, podiatrists, anesthesiologists and dentists.

You can be a CRNA in the military or private sector, working in free-standing surgical clinics, hospitals, pain clinics and in regular physicians' offices. You can practice anesthesiology under the supervision of a solo anesthesiologist, with a group or in collaboration with other surgery personnel. You may be hired by a hospital or a specific doctor or work with a team of certified nurse anesthetists. The pay is generally one of the best among nursing specialties, in excess of $160,000 per year.

CRNAs provide the sole source of anesthesia care for more than 2/3 of all rural hospitals in the US so that about 70 million individuals can have access to anesthesia care where there is a shortage of anesthesiologists to provide them care. They care for the person before, during and after anesthetic procedures, including those during the labor and delivery process.

CRNAs are responsible for continually monitoring the body functions and vital signs of a patient in surgery. The patients' lives are literally in the hands of the certified nurse anesthetist during the operative period. The anesthetist is responsible for managing the ventilator, the amount of anesthetic the patient receives and the patient's responses to anesthesia during surgery. He or she has to make critical decisions in a short period of time and must be able to quickly communicate findings with the rest of the surgical team. It is an exciting job with great pay.

Nurse Midwife
A certified nurse midwife or CNM is an optional career path you can take with a little bit of extra education. Many programs require that you have a Bachelor's degree in Nursing in order to be accepted; however, some programs simply ask that you are an RN but do not have your Bachelor's degree. In such cases, an accelerated nursing education program is provided to bring you up to the Bachelor's degree level before going on to the midwife aspect of the program.

There are two programs, essentially leading to the same job description. A CNM is a certified nurse midwife who has been a registered nurse and who has graduated from an accredited nurse midwifery program (accredited by the Accreditation Commission for Midwifery Education or ACME). They have passed the national certification exam in order to become a CNM.

A CM is a certified midwife who graduated with a Bachelor's Degree in a health field that was not a nursing education. They still need to graduate from an ACME program and take the national certification exam to become a CM. The test is put forth by the American Midwifery Certification Board (ACMB). Both CNMs and CMs take the same examination to become licensed in the field of midwifery.

As a certified nurse midwife or CNM, you provide care and reproductive counselling for women who have not yet conceived a child, for those who are pregnant, for those delivering a baby and for mothers who are in the postpartum phase of their pregnancy. Family-centered medical care is provided to women throughout their reproductive years by CNMs or CMs.
CNMs play an important role in the pregnancy and delivery of infants. They commonly reduce the necessity for high tech interventions commonly brought on by the care given by obstetricians. Certified nurse midwives have more patients and use somewhat

different techniques that have been found to reduce the number of Cesarean sections when compared to deliveries tended to by obstetricians. Even so, CNMs are trained in the same high tech scientific procedures as doctors—as they relate to pregnancy and delivery. They simply don't use them as often when caring for a mother in labor and delivery.

Certified nurse midwives attend about ten percent of all vaginal births in the US and take care of about 7 percent of all laboring mothers. A total of 97 percent of these deliveries take place in a hospital setting, while 2 percent take place in a freestanding birth center. About 1 percent of all midwife-attended deliveries take place in the home but not all CNMs will do this route of delivery for safety reasons.

CNMs don't just attend to births. In fact, only ten percent of their total work time is spent on the labor and delivery aspect of their job. Besides delivering babies, they give routine GYN examinations, do prenatal care for pregnant mothers, contraceptive and reproductive counselling, and postpartum care. Ninety percent of all patient care is directed toward preventative care medicine.

Certified nurse midwives generally work independently but work under the indirect (and sometimes direct) supervision of a physician, usually an OB/GYN physician. The supervising physician can participate in a complicated delivery and can do necessary Cesarean sections with the assistance of the midwife.

Certified nurse midwives work in many different medical settings, including freestanding birth centers, private practice clinics, hospitals, home birth organizations and regular health clinics. You are practically guaranteed to have a job available to you because of a growing need for CNMs, especially in rural or underserved areas.

Certified nurse midwives have other career options besides clinical midwifery. Besides working as a midwife in a clinical practice, you can work in administration, research, for the development of domestic and world health policy, legislation and education of other nurse midwife candidates. CNMs work in public institutions, private practice, university settings, and in hospitals geared toward military families. You can work for an HMO, set up your own home birth organization, or set up a birth center where you will work with other CNMs and CMs. Some midwives work with the poor pregnant mother in international health programs or in public health facilities, helping to improve the health of mothers and children everywhere.

The median salary for a certified nurse midwife is around $70,000 although the salary varies with where you are working and how much experience you have. Many certified nurse midwives have benefit packages associated with their job. Because you are participating in the unpredictable world of labor and delivery, your hours can be quite irregular, with deliveries happening just about any time, day or night.

Certified Nurse Practitioner
A certified nurse practitioner is generally called a "nurse practitioner" with the "C" inserted before NP to become CNP or NPC to indicate his or her certified status. These

are generally nurses who already have a four year degree and are registered nurses who complete a Master's degree equivalent in an accredited certified nurse practitioner program, which is generally up to two years additional training beyond the original four year program. Different states have different laws regarding nurse practitioner licensure. Many states require the nurse practitioner to have a Master's degree and to pass the national nurse practitioner certification examination.

Some states allow for a complete independence for the nurse practitioner and others require that prescriptive practices only be allowed by doctors with NPs working in collaboration with the doctor. There are still a few states that do not recognize nurse practitioner licensure nor do they allow nurse practitioners to work in the field independently as an NP.

Nurse practitioners work relatively independently in a variety of settings, which can include the following aspects of their job description:

> Obtaining a history, ordering tests, ordering and performing procedures, and performing a physical examination on outpatient clinical patients.

> Diagnosing, managing and treating a variety of diseases

> Writing prescriptions. Like doctors, nurse practitioners can apply to have a DEA number so that they can prescribe scheduled medications.

> Helping, through education, patients needing advice in the area of health and prevention of disease, including carrying on with healthy lifestyles.

Nurse practitioners can work in a variety of specialties and subspecialties, depending on their area of interest and background education. These can include emergency medicine, cardiology services, family practice, psychiatry, geriatrics, nephrology, neonatology, oncology, pediatrics, school health, OB/GYN, and other areas of clinical medicine.

Some nurse practitioners work in clinics without doctor supervision. Others work together with doctors as a joint health care team. Their scope of practice and authority depends on state laws. For example, some states allow nurse practitioners to write prescriptions, while other states do not.

While nurse practitioners must abide by state laws governing nurse practitioners, they are certified nationally. There is a consistent level of professional practice standards across the nation, however. This means that nurse practitioners need to be regulated at both the state and national levels.

Certification is national and is offered by means of several different national nursing organizations, including the American Nurses' Association, Psychiatric Mental Health Nurse Practitioner (PMHNP) certification, and the Pediatric Nursing Certification Board, and many others. In order to become certified in any of these areas, you need to have a Master's level degree in an accredited NP program. Most of the certification examinations involve subspecialty areas of practice, including adult nursing, acute care, pediatrics, geriatrics, women's health care, psychiatry, and family practice.

The recertification process only involves the nurse practitioner showing proof of ongoing continuing education. Because there are so many subspecialties, you will have different initials to indicate your certification after your name, including things like CNP-Peds (for a certified nurse practitioner in pediatrics, FNP-C (for a Certified Family Nurse Practitioner), or ARNP (which stands for Advanced Registered Nurse Practitioner). This involves a broader category of nurse specialists that includes certified nurse midwives, nurse anesthetists, or clinical nurse specialists.

There are a variety of other ways you can participate as a registered nurse with an advanced degree of some sort. The pathways to becoming an RN with an advanced degree are many and varied. You get to work as an RN for a period of time and/or get an advanced degree with more pay and a greater degree of independence.

If you enjoyed this book, would you be kind enough to leave a review on Amazon?

Your reviews can help others to see what kinds of helpful resources are out there!

I'll talk to you soon and see you in the next book!

Thank you and good luck on your medical endeavors!

- Chase Hassen

Nurse Superhero

Made in the USA
Lexington, KY
29 September 2016